Anti Inflammatory Diet

Simple Steps To Erase Inflammation and Become the Healthiest You

Kelvin Sprinkle

Table of Contents

Introduction

Inflammation. Just thinking of that word can make your skin crawl and your mind immediately run to the thought of infection. You probably think of the itchy, red, swollen, and pus-filled cut you got when you were seven.

However, what if you knew that inflammation can plague people without an actual injury? This is known as chronic inflammatory disease and there are several types out there that affect different aspects of the body.

This book will teach you how food can help you fight off inflammation, and keep bad flare ups at bay.

Chapter 1: What is an Anti Inflammatory Diet

An anti inflammatory diet is pretty straight forward, but there is more to it than meets the eye. While yes, it is a diet that helps reduce inflammation for people with arthritis and other complications that cause inflammation. There are many different benefits to this diet, and each one is unique in its own way.

Many people feel like a simple diet change can't fix how they feel with their physical complications. However, the truth is that it is very simple to help your pain and discomfort with nothing more than a simple diet change. While it can't completely eradicate the problems that you may have, it can drastically reduce them.

Food plays a huge role in how our bodies operate and it can dictate if you feel good or if you feel bad on a daily basis. What you need to eat depends a lot on what your body itself is like. While the fact that some people are able to eat foods that other people find drags the down may seem unfair, it is just the body chemistry and how it breaks down the food.

There is no specific diet plan that helps every single person on the planet one hundred percent, an anti inflammatory diet has proven to reduce inflammation drastically in around eighty-five percent of people, and help decrease inflammation in the other fifteen percent of people.

This diet is high in fiber, and antioxidants. This helps your body help itself. These ingredients help your body fight off inflammation in situations where you do not need the inflammation to keep yourself healthy. This diet will help you keep your inflammation in check and help you feel more in control of your body.

What Causes Inflammation

The body is a wonderful thing. It has so many different ways to fight off foreign bodies that happen to enter your bloodstream. Inflammation is actually a defense mechanism that helps your body fight off infection. Your body starts to produce more white blood cells so that the infection can be stopped. This causes inflammation.

This is generally your body's way of fighting off problems that can be serious or life-threatening. It can help your body from going into sepsis or shock from a wound that gets infected or an infection in your organs. Inflammation may be uncomfortable, but when it has a valid cause, it is absolutely necessary. You want to make sure that you are paying attention to your inflammation, however, because if it does not go away, it could be a sign of something more serious going on.

Sometimes inflammation does not have a cause and that is when you have to get checked for other problems like arthritis. Inflammation is not always helpful, because sometimes the body decides to start attacking itself for no reason. Your body seems to think that you have a problem when in reality you do not. It often happens due to the fact that your joints are not as cushioned as they used to be, and the body's reaction is to try to add that cushion with inflammation.

Signs of Inflammation

Redness: This is a common sign of inflammation. Your skin may be a strong red, or mottled red. It could also be streaky as well. But there are many people who do not have severe redness when their skin is inflamed; however, even the slightest bit of off put red should be taken note of.

Heat: An inflamed area is often warmer than the other areas of your skin. It can feel hot to the touch and also can feel like the heat is radiating up your skin from the affected area. This is a normal reaction to inflammation.

Swelling: Another normal sign of inflammation. The affected area will swell to try to keep the infection in one area. Swelling can be slightly irritating, and can make the area feel stiff and tight. This is a side effect of inflammation, and is generally one of the first lines of defense against foreign bodies in your bloodstream.

Pain: Another one of the first indicators of inflammation, this sends a signal to your brain that something hurts, and that something is not right. Your body will then usually respond to the pain with swelling and the other symptoms that come with inflammation.

Loss of function: This is something that is a bit more extreme than the other symptoms, but it is usually caused when a nerve is affected, whether it be from swelling putting pressure on that nerve, or the nerve was cut. Generally, function returns fairly quickly.

General Illness: If you feel like you are feverish or nauseous, this could be a sign of inflammation. However, if it persists and does not get better, it could be a sign of sepsis or blood poisoning, which can happen when inflammation fails to stop the spread of rapidly multiplying bacteria.

The Science Behind Inflammation

Immune cells work to fight off infection. To do this, they start the process known as inflammation. Different tissues are released such as histamine, and they force the blood vessels to expand, and allow more blood to reach the area the injury has occurred in. This causes the area to become hot and for redness to appear.

Pain and swelling are known as defense mechanisms. They make sure that you are keeping things away from the injured area to avoid hurting it more. These may be annoying, but without them, the injuries would end up getting much worse without us even trying.

Inflammation is generally a helpful line of defense when it comes to our bodies. It is meant to drive out infection, and keep us from dying. However, it is not always as helpful as we feel that it should be.

When Inflammation is Not Helpful

Unfortunately, sometimes inflammation is not very helpful. It can actually cause several chronic diseases that cause a lot of pain and discomfort. The most commonly known is Rheumatoid Arthritis. This is also known as RA. It is very unpleasant and causes the joints to be permanently inflamed.

It can also cause psoriasis, which is an inflammation of the skin. It causes red spots on the skin to appear and can make the person who has it very self-conscious. Plaque psoriasis can cause the skin to be really flaky as well. Psoriasis is not always really painful, but it can be itchy and unpleasant at times. It also is not well understood by many people, and they feel like the person with psoriasis is carrying some contagious disease like leprosy.

There are also chronic inflammation diseases of the bowels. The most commonly known is Crohn's Disease. This can cause severe stomach pain, as if the person constantly has severely bad gas. This can leave them unable to move at times, and at others, constantly feeling the need to go to the bathroom.

Another bowel inflammation disease is ulcerative colitis. This is where ulcers can literally form on the inside of the bowels, and often causes the need for a stoma so that no waste material can enter the rest of the body.

However, if you do suffer from inflammatory diseases, there is good news. The right diet can help you manage your suffering and help you get back on track with where you need to be in your life so that you can enjoy yourself more, and be in less pain and discomfort.

Chapter 2: How to Make a Great Meal Plan

The secret to having a great diet where you do not have to fight inflammation pain, is to start with meal planning. You want to make sure that you are planning your meals ahead so that you will always have the food you need to fight the inflammation that is plaguing you.

What Is Meal Planning?

Meal planning is the most important part of making sure you have a good diet. One that is balanced and full of the nutrients that you need to fight off inflammation. Most people try to just wing it as they begin a new diet, and that is how most diet changes fail to stick.

You want to make sure that when you plan a meal, you are not just planning a day or so ahead. You want to plan at least a week to a month in advance. This will keep you from having a day where you do not want to go to the store to pick up that night's dinner, and causing you to eat something that will cause your inflammation to flare up.

Meal plans do not have to be super intense and extensive. You want to make sure that you are planning healthy food and stuff that will help you rather than harm you, though. This is something that cannot be stressed enough. You want to do some research on what will help you the most and the foods that are known to fight inflammation. Otherwise, you will have a hard time making the right meal plans.

Most people develop a system, and then it gets easier to plan meals in advance. Once you find what works for you, you will be able to have the whole meal planning experience down, and you will be better off in life for the organization that you are experiencing.

Meal plans are just a tool to help you succeed, so you need to find what works for you. While you can ask a friend for advice, you do not have to adhere strictly to the advice they are trying to give you. Because what works for them may not work for you. If you are trying to use a system that does not work, then you will not be able to stick with it.

Get Inspired for Planning

The hardest part about meal planning is getting bored of eating the same foods over and over again. The secret most people don't know is that you don't have to eat the same foods over and over again. Most people just do not know a lot of recipes, so they decide that they do not want to be stuck in a rut of eating the same things each week.

Spend time on the internet, and waist deep in cookbooks. The internet is a lot easier than cookbooks, though, because you can input the ingredients that you have or that you want to use, and find a lot of recipes based on those ingredients. With a cookbook, you have to manually go through and find recipes that use the ingredients you need. If you are an adventurous sort, then maybe cookbooks are the best choice for you. Whatever you choose, make sure that you are enjoying the hunt.

You can find amazing recipes, and some will be included here, that are good for easing inflammation in the body. You want to make sure that you are finding recipes that you will like, and that you will want to keep in your recipe cycle on a regular basis. It is okay to try something out of your comfort zone, just make sure a whole week is not filled with food you are not going to like. You want to be excited for each week, and you want to feel satisfied so that you are not turning to greasy or unhealthy food that will flare your inflammation.

When you are planning your meals, you want to make sure that you are also staying within our budget. There are a lot of cellphone apps that will find the lowest price for ingredients at stores near you. This way you know where to go before you even do your shopping. Another thing that helps with meal planning is couponing. The more money you save, the better chance you have of sticking with planning your meals in advance.

Make sure you ask people in your household what they like to eat as well, and that you are not only cooking for your taste buds. Unless you live alone, then it doesn't matter, because you are the only one eating the food. However, if you have a family then you also need to plan your meals around them. Make sure to get them on board with the diet change plan so that they won't try to veer you off of a healthy diet that will reduce your pain and discomfort.

When planning, it is a good idea to get a plan on what the weather is going to be like that week in your area. That way you can have a plan for if you want a soup, or if you want a salad. You want to be sure that you are going to want to eat what you have planned that day, so being in sync with the weather always helps. However, weather can change on a dime, so it is always good to plan a few extra meals that can be weather adaptable a month.

When you find some recipes that you would like to try, you have to make sure that you save them. A lot of people plan for a meal, but then try to find the recipe that they were wanting to use, and they can't find it. Make sure that you either save it via the internet or write down the recipe and put it somewhere you can easily access it and remember where it is. This could be websites such as Pinterest, or an actual cork board if you are old fashioned. You could make your own cookbook of actual recipes, and then you will be able to access the recipes at any time. There are so many ways that you can store your ideas, it is crazy.

One way to keep track of meals that you loved, and meals that were not such a big hit, is to keep a meal journal. These are almost like a food diary, only you just notate what meals you liked and what you didn't. You can then go back when you think of using a recipe to make sure that you and your family enjoyed it, so that you don't end up making a bad dish again. You can also note what you can do differently to make it better, and add any changes that you yourself made to the meal, and that will help you with making sure that you are ending up with the same results every time. You can organize your meal journal however you like. You can set it up like a cookbook, where each meal has its own space, or you can set it up like a diary where you note the day and what meal you had. Meal journals are a helpful tool that will keep you on track with planning meals for your family.

Remember that unlike just meal planning for a big family, you should plan every meal for an anti inflammatory diet. Not just dinner. You want to plan breakfasts, lunches, and dinners for the entire family on weekends, and breakfasts and lunches for yourself on the weekdays. You want to make sure that you are all in order when you go to do the grocery shopping so that you can stay away from the junk food, and the food that is not helpful.

Helpful ways to meal plan

There are many ways to help plan your meals. Everyone is different, but here are some of the most common ways that people have found to help them plan meals for their families. If you find one on here that may work for you, then you can feel free to use it. If you find one elsewhere that works, then feel free to use that.

- Plan by the week: A lot of people plan in week-long increments. They take one day of the week every week that they can spend time shopping, and they go to the store and use a list of ingredients that they need to find what they want to buy for the week. This is a great idea so that you can be sure to use everything that you buy, however, it can get a little more expensive in the long run because you are less likely to need to buy in bulk.

- Plan by the Month: This is something people do when they get paid every two weeks, or they get paid every month. It is also a great money saver because then you can buy supplies in bulk, and not have a problem with having too much waste because it doesn't get used in time. You can find great deals and do a lot of shopping at once, to cut down on those hassling runs to the supermarket. Instead of going four times a month, you only need to go once. This also helps save in gas.

- Make a calendar: you can buy a typical calendar, or get one for free from your local bank, and use that to notate what you are going to have each day. This will help give you a visual reference so that you do not have to remember a million meals for a month. You want to make sure that you get a calendar that has the big day squares so that you can fit all of your meals for the day in the blanks.

- Get a chalkboard: If you are tired of hearing "mom, what's for dinner" a million times, then you should get a chalk or white board that can help you show your family what is for dinner. Write the day's meals down each night. It will also help you remember, so you can just check the fridge or wherever you hang the board and see what you need to set out for your meals that day.

- Paper list: This is for the people who have to see the everything on paper to really feel like things are set in stone. A paper list is just like having a chalkboard only you can fit several days of meals on it so that you can pull out meat to defrost a few days before if you need to. It is also easier to adhere to the meals if you see them several days in advance so that you can prepare for the prep that they may need, and possibly do it in advance on a day where you are making an easier meal.

- Use an app: There are several apps out there that have been created for meal planning. A good one is recipe keeper for android. It has a place to store recipes, shopping lists, and even your meal plans. You can look at it to see what you need to make that day, and it is all in one space, so you don't have to bog your phone down with a lot of apps. You can search for a meal planning app that works for you and your phone.

Meal planning is very important, as it will help you keep on track with your diet. If you do not plan your meals, it is a lot easier to fall prey to the convenient and easy junk food. You want to stay away from that so that you do not have really bad flare-ups. Cause junk food and foods that are high in trans fats have been known to cause inflammation flare ups.

Chapter 3: Recipe Book

This chapter will be full of recipes for meals that will help you reduce inflammation and get back to living your life. There will be meals for breakfast, lunch, and dinner. Along with snacks and desserts, this will be a complete starter cookbook for you so that you can get an idea of what you should be eating. The end of this chapter will have foods that you should eat so that you can look for your own recipes, or even create your own.

Breakfasts

There is not much online about breakfast recipes because it seems most meal plans center around dinners that you can serve your family. However, this book will give you a few starter ideas if you are stumped after an extensive internet search. These delicious recipes will spark your taste buds, but not your inflammation. You will want to have these for every meal, but remember, there are other recipes out there as well.

Vegetable Scramble Wrap

What you need

- Egg substitute (¾ cup per serving)

- Chopped green bell pepper (2 tablespoons per serving)

- Chopped red onion (2 tablespoons per serving)

- Whole wheat tortilla (1 ten inch per serving)

- Minced garlic (to taste- optional)

In a nonstick skillet coated with cooking spray, cook the bell pepper, onion, (and garlic if used) until soft. Add the egg substitute, and cook until the egg is set. Spoon the ingredients into a tortilla, and serve hot.

This is great coupled with a light Greek yogurt, or a side of fruit While this is great alone, it is important to have a balanced meal, and you want to have some dairy or fruit. Make sure that you are drinking water, rather than soda or harsh juices. A one hundred percent juice may help, though. Stay away from high acidic juices if you have Crohn's disease or ulcerative colitis.

Granola with Oven Dried Strawberries

Oven dried strawberries are delicious alone, but they are not very balanced for your diet. You want to make sure that you are eating balanced for breakfast, because it is the most important meal of the day, and you want to give your brain the power it needs to function.

This takes some time to make so you may want to make it the night before and store it in an airtight container. This is a big recipe and makes ten to twelve servings so that you can use it for breakfast, or as a side, or even a nice snack. You can also use it as dessert toppings as well. This stores well, so you do not have to worry about it going bad in a short amount of time. The reason is that you are removing all of the moisture from the food so it won't mold or go stale. As long as it is stored in an airtight container, it can last for quite a while.

What you need

- 2 ½ cups of raw almonds. Unsalted with no artificial flavors.
- 2 cups of macadamia nuts
- 1 ½ cups of coconut flakes
- 6 dried apricots
- 10 medium strawberries
- 2/3 cups of dried cranberries
- 2/3 cups of chia seeds. (Yes what you used to use to make chia pets. The seeds are really good for you and full of antioxidants)
- 2/3 cup dried goji berries.

First, you have to dry the strawberries. This takes the longest amount of time as it has to be done slowly to keep from ruining the strawberries or burning them. First, you have to wash dry and slice the strawberries. You want to slice them thinly and lengthwise. Make sure to chop off the very top of the strawberry. You should get around five slices from each strawberry.

Spray a pan that has holes with no-stick cooking spray. (I find a pizza pan designed for thin crispy crusts works wonders. You want to make sure that you spread them out in a single layer so they can all dry properly. Put the strawberries in an oven that has been preheated to 160 degrees, and cook for one and a half hours. Take them out, flip them over, and put them back in for another one and a half hours.

Once you remove the strawberries, turn your oven up to 300 degrees and then move the strawberries in a bowl to cool. Once the oven has reached temp, put the macadamia nuts and almonds on a baking tray and roast for ten minutes. Make sure you stir them quite often. About once a minute, and pay special attention at the end so they do not burn and stick. When they are golden, remove them to a bowl to cook.

On the same baking tray, place the coconut flakes on it, and put in the oven for two minutes to roast. While they are roasting, throw the nuts in the food processor to chunk them up a bit more.

Mix all of the ingredients together, and let cool completely. Once completely cooled, put in an airtight container to store what you are not going to eat at that time.

To Eat:

You can eat this as a cereal. It is very delicious with a soy or almond milk over the top of it. You can use it to top many desserts, and you can use it on greek yogurt. Serve as a side to eggs to skip the boring eggs and toast routine. Mix in some peanut butter and make drop cookies with it. This is very versatile, and you will find that it makes a great side to many dishes, along with a great breakfast itself.

Berry and Whole Grain Waffles

What You Need

- 2 eggs (or egg substitute), beaten
- 1 ¾ cup of skim milk
- ¼ cup of canola oil
- ¼ cup unsweetened applesauce
- 1 tsp of vanilla extract
- 1 ¼ cup of whole wheat pastry flour
- ½ cup flaxseed meal
- ¼ cup wheat germ
- 1 cup of mixed berries (or your favorite berries)
- 4 tsp baking powder
- 1 tbsp sugar
- ¼ tsp salt

In a large bowl, whisk together milk, eggs, oil, applesauce, and vanilla extract.

Slowly beat in all dry ingredients aside from berries until smooth.

Once smooth, add berries, and mix well.

Preheat waffle iron coated with cooking spray, and add batter. Cook until crispy and golden, then enjoy. Top with fat-free whipped cream. Make sure it is not made with hydrogenated oils, though. A good choice is homemade whipped cream or Reddi Whip. Add additional berries if so desired.

Avocado toast and egg

What You Need

- One slice of whole wheat bread (2 slices if making a sandwich)

- ½ tsp of ghee

- ½ an avocado, sliced

- Fresh spinach to taste (about a handful)

- 1 egg poached (scrambled works as well)

- Red pepper flakes to taste.

Toast bread and top with ghee

place the sliced avocado, and spinach on top of the ghee. Top with eggs, and garnish with red pepper flakes.

Enjoy open with knife and fork, or add second piece of toast to make a sandwich.

This is a pretty balanced breakfast right here. You might add a side of fruit or yogurt, but if you don't, it is not the end of the world because this is a really good balance of nutrients for breakfast.

Chia Quinoa Porridge

What You Need

- 1 cup of cashew milk. Thick is best

- 2 cups of cooked quinoa

- 1 cup of fresh blueberries

- ¼ cup of toasted walnuts

- ½ tsp ground cinnamon

- 2 tsp raw honey (agave works too)

- 1 tbsp chia seeds

Combine cashew milk and quinoa in a sauce pan, and heat slowly over medium high heat.

Add the berries, walnuts, and cinnamon, and heat till all is warm. Remove from heat and stir in honey. Top with chia seeds and enjoy.

You can serve this as a side to an egg, but this is pretty balanced by itself.

Breakfast Pizza

Yes, that is correct. Don't skip over this recipe and scoff at it. A breakfast pizza can be tasty and it can be good for helping reduce inflammation at the same time. You want to make sure that your ingredients are healthy, and from there you can enjoy pizza. Here is a recipe for a delicious breakfast pizza that will make you look forward to breakfast again.

What You Need

- 1 cup of oat flour, or gluten free flour

- ½ cup of ground flaxseed

- ½ cup of water (or more if this is not enough to completely moisten the batter)

- 1 cup of scrambled egg substitute

- ¼ cup crisped turkey bacon crumbled (bout three strips

- ½ cup goat cheese

Mix well, and spread onto a pizza pan. Crust should only be about one centimeter thick. Bake in an oven preheated to 350 degrees for twenty minutes. Once the crust is finished, top with goat cheese, egg substitute scrambled, and crisp turkey bacon. Stick back in the oven and cook for another five minutes, or until cheese has melted.

These recipes are very good to help start your day off without inflammation. You want to make sure that you have plenty of good breakfasts that are anti inflammatory, otherwise, you will turn back to the packaged breakfasts, or worse, skip it all together. If you have a busy morning scheduled, perhaps make something like a scrambled burrito or pizza and heat it back up in the morning. Make sure that you eat breakfast every day, and that you are eating a balanced breakfast as well. A lot of these are okay to eat alone, however, some may need a supplement which will be noted on the recipe.

Another good breakfast food is the smoothie. Next, we will go over some anti inflammatory smoothie. These are good when you are on the move, and don't have time to sit down and eat a balanced meal. Instead of eating it, you can drink it, and you will still have a balanced meal for breakfast.

Smoothies

Here are some recipes for smoothies to help you on days when you are running behind and still need breakfast. If you don't have time for a sit-down meal, then you can take your meal to go and eat it through a straw. There are smoothies that can be made for dinners and lunches as well, but we are going to fixate on breakfast smoothies because breakfast is the most common skipped meal a day.

Healthy Dried Strawberry Oat Smoothie

What You Need

¼ cup chia seeds

¼ cup flaxseed

¼ cup oats

¼ cup strawberries

¼ cup strawberry yogurt

Pinch of Kale

Pinch of Spinach

ice

Dried Strawberries to taste

Mix all ingredients but the dried strawberries in a blender. Blend until smooth. Make sure that there are no big oats or seeds to avoid choking, so you will want to blend for a good forty-five seconds before you stop the blender and serve in a glass. Top with dried strawberries and enjoy. You can also top with a fat-free whipped cream to add an extra pop of sweetness.

Acai Cacao Smoothie

This is a really healthy smoothie that will make you feel like you are indulging in a naughty treat, only you will not have to deal with any inflammation flare-ups later. You want to make sure that you enjoy this smoothie to the fullest because chocolate is seen as a no-no for inflammation, when in reality natural cacao is a great inflammation reducer.

What You Need

1 cup of coconut water

•¼ of an avocado

•1/3 cup of yogurt

•1/2 cup of fresh / frozen strawberries

•1 tablespoon of almond butter or a handful of raw almonds

•1 tablespoon of goji berries (blended or sprinkled on top)

•1 tablespoon of cacao powder

•1/2 tablespoon of cacao nibs (blended or sprinkled on top)

•1 teaspoon of chia seeds

•1 teaspoon of bee pollen

•1 teaspoon of acai powder

•1/4 teaspoon of cinnamon

•A dash of Himalayan salt/sea salt

•A little honey, maple syrup, or stevia natural sweetener (optional)

Blend in a high-speed blender for around forty-five seconds. This will ensure that all the chunks are smoothed out. You will not want to put this smoothie down and will miss it when it's gone. You can also add protein powder to balance it out more. Coconut flakes in this are really good as well. Top with dried strawberries if you wish.

Blueberry Chocolate Spirulina Smoothie

What You Need

1 cup milk of choice (I used raw milk)

•1/3 avocado

•1/2 cup fresh or frozen blueberries

•1 tablespoon tahini

•1 tablespoon cacao powder

•1/2 tablespoon cacao nibs (blend some and sprinkle some on top)

•1/2 tablespoon spirulina

•1/4 teaspoon vanilla powder or extract

•1/2 tablespoon honey to sweeten (substitute maple syrup or stevia)

1 serving of your preferred protein powder

•1/2 cup fresh or frozen strawberries

•1 cup spinach, kale, or other leafy green

•1 tablespoon flax or chia seeds

Mix these all together in your blender for thirty seconds, and serve. You will love this smoothie, and even though the ingredients may seem odd, it tastes like heaven, and you will want to have it for every meal. It is cautioned against that because you want to make sure that you are eating other foods as well. Okay, maybe you won't go that far, but this is a really good smoothie, and again, it's got chocolate.

Blood Orange and Kefir Smoothie

Kefir is a fermented milk and is not for everyone. It is quite sour tasting, but if you like goats milk, it tastes quite similar, however, you can substitute nut milk or raw milk if you do not feel that kefir is for you. A blood orange is much like a grapefruit, only much smaller, and not as sour in taste. They can be hard to find, but most Whole Food stores should have them. Now onto the smoothie.

What You Need

1 cup of kefir (substitute nut milk or raw milk)

•2 small to medium blood oranges, peeled (substitute regular oranges)

½ teaspoon of vanilla extract or powder

•½ tablespoon of cacao powder

•½ tablespoon of coconut oil

•½ of an avocado

•½ cup of raspberries, strawberries, blueberries, blackberries, or any other berry

You want to blend this a little longer because oranges do not like to break down well. Blend this smoothie for a good fifty seconds to get that silky smooth texture. This is a great smoothie, but it's not entirely balanced. Add a piece of toast or a bagel to get some grains in your smoothie, or add some flaxseed into the smoothie.

Here are some smoothies that will help you get a good start on your day and help you get a head start on your inflammation.

You can also have these as a snack even if you had a great breakfast. These are very versatile, and you can take them wherever. Great for days where the carpool time just does not allow for breakfast in the traditional manner. Just a minute or so and you are ready to go.

Next up are lunches that are anti inflammatory. Some people try to skip lunch, and while it is not as insanely important as breakfast, it is important to eat right to stay on top of your inflammation, and that means eating lunch as well. These lunches are pretty easy to pack for the next day and take with you to work or to school. Wherever you may need to be with your lunch. Just make sure your lunchbox has utensils. You will want to tell everyone about these lunches, and you won't even notice how healthy are. While other people are feeding their bodies things that would hurt yours, they will be envying your delicious, and nutritious lunch that keeps your body in movement mode.

Spinach, Goat Cheese, and Red Bell Pepper Salad (With Oregano Dressing)

What You Need

2 tablespoons of extra-virgin olive oil

2 tablespoons of fresh lemon juice

1 tablespoon of chopped fresh oregano

4 cups of (packed) baby spinach leaves, coarsely chopped (about 4 ounces)

1 1/2 large red bell peppers, diced

1 1/2 cups of diced celery (about 3 stalks)

3/4 cup of crumbled soft fresh goat cheese

1/3 cup of chopped red onion

This is pretty easy to make because all you have to do really is make the dressing and then mix the other ingredients in together. To make the dressing, whisk together the first three ingredients, and then salt and pepper to taste (Make sure to use sea salt). Then add the last five ingredients and enjoy your salad. You can keep your dressing and salad separate until you are ready to eat in order to avoid having a soggy lunch come lunch time. This makes four servings, so you can share it with your family.

Citrus and Ginger Yogurt Salad

What You Need

1 pink grapefruit, peeled

2 large tangerines or Minneolas, peeled

3 navel oranges

1/2 cup dried cranberries

2 tablespoons honey

1/4 teaspoon ground cinnamon

1 16- or 17.6-ounce container Greek yogurt

2/3 cup minced crystallized ginger

1/4 cup golden brown sugar

Additional dried cranberries

Break the grapefruit and tangerines into sections. Take those sections and cut into thirds. Cut the white part of the oranges off (known as the pith) and then cut them the same as the grapefruit and tangerines. Mix in the dried cranberries, ground cinnamon, and honey. Chill at least an hour. While that is chilling, mix the ginger and yogurt in a separate bowl, and let that chill. When ready to serve, spoon yogurt on the fruit and top with brown sugar and cranberries.

Pan Seared Salmon on a Bed of Baby Arugula Salad

This can be made as a dinner, and then the leftovers can be used for lunch. Or you can make it for lunch the night before, just leave the dressing off of the salad, and keep the salad in an airtight container until ready to consume. Salmon can be consumed hot or cold.

What You Need

2 center-cut salmon fillets (6 oz. each)

1 1/2 Tbsp fresh lemon juice

1 1/2 Tbsp olive oil

Salt and freshly ground black pepper, to taste

For the salad:

3 cups baby arugula leaves

2/3 cup grape or cherry tomatoes, halved

1/4 cup thinly slivered red onion

Salt and freshly ground black pepper, to taste

1 Tbsp extra-virgin olive oil

1 Tbsp red-wine vinegar

First, you must marinate the salmon, with some delicious seasonings. This will give it a great flavor to complement the arugula salad. In a shallow bowl, toss the fillets with Lemon juice, olive oil, pepper and salt to taste. A dash of lemon pepper and minced garlic is also very tasty when added.

Heat a skillet on high and coat in nonstick spray. Place the fillets skin-side up, and cook for two to three minutes shaking and moving the fish to keep the fish from sticking to the pan.

Turn the heat down to medium, and cover the pan. Cook the salmon for another four minutes, until it is medium rare, and the skin is crisp.

Combine the salad ingredients, and then drizzle with olive oil and vinegar and top with salt and pepper to taste when ready to serve. Enjoy!.

Roasted Root Vegetables

You can make extra of these as a side for dinner, and take the extra for lunch the next day. This is a great source of nutrients and is so tasty, everyone will be begging for your recipe.

What You Need

1 2 1/2-pound butternut squash, peeled, seeded, cut into 1/2-inch pieces (about 5 cups)

1 1/2 pounds Yukon Gold potatoes, unpeeled, cut into 1/2-inch pieces

1 bunch beets (about 1 1/2 pounds), trimmed but not peeled, scrubbed, cut into 1/2-inch pieces

1 medium-size red onion, cut into 1/2-inch pieces (about 2 cups)

1 large turnip, peeled, cut into 1/2-inch pieces (about 1 cup)

1 head of garlic, cloves separated, peeled

2 tablespoons olive oil

Preheat your oven to 425 degrees and grease up two large baking pans. Evenly spread out the veggies amongst both pans, and season to taste. Cook for a little over an hour, stirring occasionally. Eat warm or cold with a side of mild hummus.

Curried Chicken Salad, Spiced Chickpeas, and Raita

This is an interesting Indian style dish that will get your taste buds dancing, and most likely you dancing too, knowing you can eat this deliciousness, and not have a flare up. Food this delicious needs to be shared with the world. Bring a little extra for your coworkers to try. This makes four servings.

What You Need

1 medium onion, chopped (1 cup)

1 tablespoon minced garlic

1 tablespoon minced peeled ginger

2 tablespoons vegetable oil

1 tablespoon curry powder

1 teaspoon ground cumin

2 medium tomatoes, chopped (1 cup)

1 cup plain yogurt

2 tablespoons cilantro

1 rotisserie chicken, meat coarsely shredded (3 to 4 cups)

1 cup red grapes, halved

For chickpeas:

1 tablespoon vegetable oil

1 (19-ounce) can chickpeas, rinsed, drained, and patted dry (2 cups)

1 teaspoon ground cumin

1/2 teaspoon turmeric

1/4 teaspoon cayenne

For raita and topping:

1 cup plain yogurt

1 seedless cucumber, peeled, cored, and chopped (2 cups)

2 tablespoons chopped mint

1/2 cup sliced almonds, toasted

Equipment:

4 (16-ounce) wide jars or containers with lids

This is a little bit of an extensive process, so it is best to make it the night before and take it for lunch the next day. You can heat it up in the microwave with no problem; just make sure to add a cup of water with a toothpick as well to make sure that you don't dry it out.

For The Chicken Salad

Cook the ginger, garlic, onion, and oil in a large skillet over medium to low heat for about five minutes, or until it is all softened. Add the curry and the cumin, and cook for another two minutes.

Add tomatoes and cook on medium-high heat until sauce is thickened, or around five minutes. Transfer to a bowl and stir in chicken, yogurt, and cilantro. Let cool.

To Make Chickpeas

Heat the oil in a cleaned skillet over medium-high heat until it shimmers, then cook the chickpeas, stirring, for 1 minute. Add cumin, turmeric, cayenne, and 1/4 teaspoon salt and cook, stirring to coat, until skillet is dry, for about 2 minutes. Cool to room temperature.

To Make Raita

Stir together yogurt, cucumber, mint, and 1/2 teaspoon salt.

To Assemble Jars

Divide the grapes between the jars, layer the chickpeas, raita, and curried chicken, and then top with almonds.

These are some tasty lunches that will leave you excited for that midday break. You will want to sneak a taste early, but promise, the wait is so worth it. These lunches will not interact with your body in a way that causes you to have to deal with flare-ups. You will love these meals, and not be afraid of them.

Next up are some dinners that will help you finish your night off without much of a problem so that you can sleep with ease, and less pain. You will love these meals, and so will your family, and friends if they visit. You will most likely want to take any leftovers for lunch the next day. Go right ahead! If you are planning a recipe that serves more people than are in your family, plan to take it for lunch the next day, and enjoy it.

Dinners

Dinner is the last meal before you go to bed. The hardest part about inflammation is it likes to really hit at night, making sleep a major difficulty. These meals will help reduce inflammation so that you can sleep easy. While you may have dessert afterward, dinner is the last actual meal that you have, so it will last longer in your body than dessert, due to the fact that it is denser and larger.

Here are some dinners that will not cause your chronic disease to flare up and cause you problems with sleeping. Caution, you will not be able to get enough of these and want to have them regularly. Enjoy them.

White Bean and Blanca Chicken Chilli

What You Need

1 pound chicken tenders or boneless, skinless chicken breasts

2 tablespoons extra-virgin olive oil

l 1 medium onion, diced

2 garlic cloves

2 15-ounce cans white or great northern beans, drained and rinsed

1 cup corn kernels, fresh or frozen and thawed

1 4-ounce can chopped green chilies

2 teaspoons ground cumin

2 teaspoons pure chili powder

1/8 teaspoon cayenne pepper

3 cups water

2 cups grated Monterey Jack cheese

2 tablespoons fresh cilantro, chopped

Season the chicken pieces with salt and pepper to taste, and then place in a large saucepan with oil heated on high. Cook for two to three minutes, or until the chicken is browned.

Lowering the heat to medium, add onion and garlic, and cook for five to six more minutes. Add the rest of the ingredients aside from the cheese, and bring to a boil. Reduce heat and simmer for about an hour. Top with cheese and cilantro.

Serve and enjoy.

Curried Potatoes with Poached Egg

What You Need

2 russet potatoes (about 2 lbs.)

1-inch fresh ginger

2 cloves garlic

1 Tbsp olive oil

2 Tbsp curry powder (hot or mild)

1 15oz. can tomato sauce

4 large eggs

½ bunch fresh cilantro (optional)

Wash the potatoes well, before you cut them into ¾-inch cubes. Place the cubed potatoes into a large pot and cover an inch over the potatoes with water. Cover the pot with a lid and then bring it up to a boil over a high heat. Boil the potatoes for about 5-6 minutes, or until they are tender when pierced with a fork. Drain the cooked potatoes in a colander.

While the potatoes are boiling, it is time to begin the sauce. Peel the ginger root with a vegetable peeler or you can scrape the skin off with the side of a spoon. Use a small holed cheese grater to grate off about one inch of ginger (less if you prefer a more subtle ginger flavor). Then, mince the garlic.

Add the ginger, garlic, and the olive oil to a large and deep skillet (or a wide based pot). Sauté the ginger and garlic over medium to low heat for 1-2 minutes, or just until they are soft and fragrant. Add the curry powder to the skillet and then sauté for about a minute more to toast the spices.

Add the tomato sauce in to the skillet and then stir to combine. Turn the heat up to medium heat and heat the sauce through. Taste the sauce and salt, if needed. Add the cooked and drained potatoes in to the skillet and then stir to coat in the sauce. Add a couple tablespoons of water if the mixture seems dry or slightly pasty.

Create four small wells into the potato mixture and then crack an egg into each well. Place a lid over the skillet and let it come to a simmer. Simmer the eggs that you cracked in the sauce for about 6-10 minutes, or until cooked through (less time if runny yolks are desired). Top with chopped fresh cilantro to taste.

Sweet Potato Frittata With a Tomato Salsa

What you Need

1 large sweet potato, about 7-8 ounces
1 tablespoon olive oil
1 shallot, peeled and minced
Sea salt
Black pepper
4 large eggs
Small handful of chives, finely snipped
8 ounces vine-ripened plum tomatoes
2 green onions, trimmed and thinly sliced on the diagonal
Handful of cilantro leaves, chopped
Juice of 1/2 lemon
3 tablespoons extra-virgin olive oil
1 tablespoon sesame oil
Dash of Tabasco sauce
Pinch of sugar (optional)
For the salsa:

To make the salsa, roughly chop the tomatoes and place them in a food processor. Add in all of the remaining ingredients and blend well, seasoning to your taste with salt and pepper, and a pinch of sugar if you like. Set aside.

For the frittata:

Heat your broiler to the highest setting.

Peel the sweet potato and then cut it into ½-inch cubes. Heat a pan suitable for the broiler, coat in cooking spray and then add in the olive oil.

When oil is hot, put in the potato and the shallot, seasoning well with salt and pepper to taste. Cook over a medium heat, turning often, for about 4-5 minutes or until potatoes are just tender and are lightly golden at the edges.

Beat the eggs lightly in a bowl, until frothy, add the chives, and pour over the sweet potatoes. Shake the pan gently and distribute the ingredients. Cook over a low heat, without stirring, for about five minutes or until the eggs begin to set at the bottom and around the sides.

Place the pan under the hot broiler for a couple of minutes until the top of the frittata has set. Be sure not to overcook the eggs or they will become rubbery. Let stand for a minute, then run a spatula around the sides of the pan and turn the frittata over onto a large plate.

Spoon the tomato salsa into a neat pile on top and serve immediately.

Here have been some tasty ideas for dinners that you can have and that you and your family will enjoy. You may have to work with the portions to find what fits your family. Happy cooking!

Chapter 4: Tips for getting rid of inflammatory problems

Along with diet and exercise, you want to know tips to help ease and possibly get rid of inflammation. The bad news is, you may never be able to completely get rid of inflammation. You may still have some discomfort some days. However, the good news is, you can drastically reduce the amount of days that happens and the severity of the inflammation as well. Your doctor will be amazed at how well you are doing if you follow these tips.

Some of these tips may need some tweaking to help you specifically, but with some adjustment, they will have you up and moving again in no time. Take your life back. The first step is to try, and while you may feel cautious about ever getting back to normal, you can certainly try.

Eat Better:

Obviously, the first step is to eat a better diet than what you are currently consuming. If you are consuming junk food on a daily basis, that could be part of what got you here in the first place. Especially so with bowel-related inflammation, but even skin and joint inflammation could have been motivators, as well. Because fast food makes your skin excrete more oils, which your body is not used to, so it causes psoriasis. Also, being bogged down with greasy foods will cause fat buildup which will make you not want to move, and that pressure that is now on your joints will cause the arthritis.

So change your diet to a healthy one. Avoid super fatty food, or foods high in bad calories. These are foods that are high in carbs and sugars and trans fats. Avoid fast food, and switch to home cooked meals. Try to go for fresh foods and vegetables so that you know what you are putting in your body. You want to try to stay away from things full of preservatives, such as boxed sauces, pasta, and frozen meals.

Instead, start making your own pasta, meals, and sauces. You will also be able to control how it tastes exactly, so you can find something that suits your taste buds exactly.

With a healthier diet, you can really help ease all of the foreign chemicals masquerading as food, that enter your blood stream and cause your body to attack itself.

Exercise:

Moving around may seem like an impossibility when you are going through a flare up, but exercise helps your body sweat, which will trick your body into thinking that it is removing the foreign entity that doesn't exist at all. This will help you ease your flare-ups. You do not have to do a lot of vigorous exercise while you are in a flare up, but you should at least do some cardio.

When you are not in a flare up, you should do your best to get in some pretty intense workouts so you can help prevent a flare-up in the future. The more you exercise, the more your body will think that things are getting better. Especially if you have rheumatoid arthritis, exercise can be very helpful. It will keep your joints moving so that they do not get stiff which will trigger the inflammation to get worse. You want to keep moving. You even want to sweat more with psoriasis. Sweating with healthy nutrients in your sweat will help reduce your symptoms on your skin as well.

If you are a person who things exercise rhymes too much with extra fries for any sort of motivation, you just need a few days at the gym. You will be able to start getting hooked on the endorphins that will flood your body from the exercise, and then you will want to move constantly. All it takes is a sincere effort, and a commitment to stick with it. Before you know it, you will be able to get active without having to psych yourself up thirty minutes beforehand.

Start small with your exercise, and you will find that things get a lot easier for you. If you try to start with an Insanity workout, you will just be setting yourself up for failure. Instead, start with some simple workouts to keep yourself in the groove, and up it from there.

Drink Green Tea:

You may think this falls under eat better, but while it could, there is so much more to green tea than it just being a beverage. It is a lot better than that. Green tea is almost like a miracle worker, due to its healing properties. It is also really good for relaxing your body so that you are not uptight.

When drinking green tea, you can drink it hot, or you can drink it cold. You should drink it cold before a workout, to prepare your muscles for the energy they are going to need, and you should drink it hot after a workout to help your muscles relax after a workout, so that you do not end up tearing anything, or being really sore because your muscles won't relax.

Green tea is a healthier alternative to pain medication as well, as it too can numb the pain receptors in your brain. You want to make sure that you are drinking it like you would take the pain pills. One cup every four hours as needed for pain.

Some people claim that the Green tea pain reducer idea is just a placebo, but even if it is, why not let it work rather than putting harmful things in your body that could potentially cause more flare-ups in the future. Just drink it and believe it works.

Green tea has antioxidants that help your body fight off the free radicals that cause inflammation and help you detox your body from bad chemicals. This will help reduce your flare-ups, as it removes the chemicals that start your body attacking itself in the first place. Green tea coupled with a good diet and exercise can really help nearly cure your flare-ups because your body will thank you for cleaning out the toxins that are weighing it down.

Green tea can help keep your body from attacking itself, so even if you did not fancy yourself a tea drinker, it may be worth it to start drinking green tea. You can also find green tea pills, but they may have other additives that nullify the effects of a cup of green tea.

Heat up a cup and enjoy the feeling. Have yourself a little tea party if you fancy, and add a nice healthy snack along with your tea to make it more interesting. Drink it hot with meals to help aid in proper digestion to avoid bowel inflammation, and to help your food do what it needs to do. Drink it cold when you are just needing a beverage and don't want to reach for a soda or a water.

Tea will help your body in more ways than just inflammation as well. It will help you lose weight as well as fight inflammation. This can help your inflammation a lot as well because there will be less fat build up in your body so that you can truly have a free body. The benefits are great.

Positive Thinking/Affirmations

This may seem really silly, but the truth is, it is not as silly as you may think. Most people underestimate the power a thought can do, but in reality, it can do quite a lot. It can change your entire outlook on things, and help you really see life in a new light. It can take you from depressed to a good mood with just a few good thoughts. It can take you from pained to feeling good just by telling your brain things are okay. You can go from stressed to carefree just by changing your thoughts from negative to positive.

There are several ways that you can change your way of thinking. You can just wake up every day and think about one thing that you like about yourself, and one thing you will do to get better. You can stop yourself from thinking negative thoughts when they happen. You can vow to think more positive thoughts a day, or you can say positive affirmations.

Affirmations seem to be the most effective, because they are easy to say, can be said in your head, and really change your train of thought before it even starts to go bad. You want to keep yourself from thinking negative thoughts, and more importantly, you want to believe them. You want to make sure that you are not just saying things positive, you have to truly be positive. At first, it may be hard, and there may be a few "fake it till you make it" scenarios, but the more you do it, the better you will find that your mind has become. Your thoughts will be easier to keep positive.

When you start saying positive affirmations, look for lists that you can start with. Eventually you will be able to make your own, but for now there are plenty of positive affirmation lists out there that will help you with how you think about your inflammation. Compile a list of about a hundred. Cycle through these each week, write them on post-it notes and stick them around your room, say them during a time of meditation. There are so many ways you can incorporate affirmations into your life.

Once you have learned how to incorporate affirmations into your life, it will get easier to say them whenever you have some downtime, or whenever you feel that you are getting too stressed.

Here are some tips that will help you handle your inflammation outside of the diet. You want to make sure that you work these tips into your life, rather than working your life around these tips because doing that will cause you to fall back to your old ways and the pain of inflammation. Again, adapt these tips as you please, and feel free to add your own tips to supplement these ones here.

Chapter 5: Success Stories

Here are some success stories from people who have tried this and have found that it works. You will want to read these if you need a little inspiration, or if you are feeling skeptical about the whole "diet changing your life" concept that this book is trying to convince you of. These people suffer from problems like ulcerative colitis, plaque psoriasis, and rheumatoid arthritis. They are normal everyday people, they are not celebrities, therefore only their first name and last initial will be revealed. Enjoy these stories, and hopefully, you find the inspiration you are looking for to begin a new life and battle inflammation with success.

Vera R.

Vera is a woman who struggles with rheumatoid arthritis, and it has plagued her for over twenty years. She is a grandmother who wanted to enjoy her grandchildren well into her older years, but arthritis has made that hard for her. She found that she could not chase kids around like she could in her younger years. Keeping up with her grandkids when they went to the park was often painful, and more times than not, she found herself sitting on a bench, just watching, rather than joining her beautiful grandbabies in play.

Finally, Vera decided that she needed a life change. She needed to be able to play with her young grandchildren before they all grew up. However, no doctor had a solution, and medication only went so far. Sadly, she watched as her grandchildren grew up and became adults, but she got her chance when her first great-grandchild was born. She searched the internet for a solution and found that many people had a lot of success by changing their diets. Vera searched her cabinets and realized that the food she made could be affecting her more than she realized. So she decided to make a change.

She changed her diet and began to start mild exercise. She found that within a month she had already begun to see results. She had more energy and fewer flare-ups. She could sleep better, and wake up feeling refreshed. She had more energy to play with her great grandkids, and take her dogs on walks and to the dog park.

Now Vera wonders why she didn't see the light before, but now that she has, she says she never wants to go back.

Kevin P.

Kevin is a young man who has suffered nearly his entire life with ulcerative colitis. He was diagnosed at the age of five. That was twenty years ago. He found that the condition affected his life quite a bit. He had to have a stoma by the time he was thirteen. This really put a damper on his social life, because his life revolved around his painful flare-ups, along with knowing where the nearest bathroom was. He tried not to let it affect him, but unfortunately, it affected him a lot. He missed a lot of school due to pain when he was growing up.

This trend followed him into adulthood. Often times, Kevin found himself in too much pain to go to work, and he found it hard to keep a job because he had to take so many sick days. He says he could have gotten disability, but that just was not him. He wanted to live a normal life and get a good job. He wanted to make sure that he got to a place in life where he could live a semi-normal life, and not have to deal with the flare-ups, or at least not as bad.

When his friend told him about an anti inflammatory diet plan, he jumped right on it, because he had nothing to lose. He started eating less inflammatory foods, and found that he had fewer flare-ups, and eventually was able to go months without a single one, and the rare times he had them, they were not as severe as they had been, and he could still function.

Since that day, he has found a good job and risen to the manager position. He loves that he is making more money, and able to support himself without disability, and can lead a normal life, just like any other male in his mid-twenties.

Carol M.

Carol is a middle-aged woman with psoriasis. It affects her arms the worst, and she often finds that it is hard to wear anything with short sleeves, because people stare, and they treat her like she has leprosy. She often found herself wearing long sleeves, even in the summer, and she hated how hot she always had to be to cover her psoriasis.

Well, one day, she learned how a change in diet could help her get better. She started following this diet plan and found many delicious recipes that she could enjoy without causing flare-ups. Since then she has bought more short sleeve shirts and is not scared to go out in public without sleeves.

Hopefully, these success stories help motivate you to try this. You can't win if you don't even try, so at least give it a shot. Who knows, you might love it.

Chapter 6: List of anti inflammatory foods

Now you can make your own recipes if you just knew what foods were good for this diet. Fret not, this chapter lists a lot of foods that are good for this diet, so that you can begin concocting your own culinary masterpieces.

Bok Choy

Green Leafy vegetables such as kale and spinach

Celery

Broccoli

Beets

Blueberries

Salmon

Pineapple

Bone Broth

Walnuts

Chia seeds

Coconut oil

Turmeric

Flaxseeds

Ginger

These foods help you with an anti inflammatory diet. Look for things that are high in omega threes and low in saturated fats.

Conclusion

Inflammation can cause a lot of problems in your life; however, it is not the end of the world if you are diagnosed with a chronic inflammatory disease. There still hope for a relatively normal life, with food, and your medication, you can go back to business as usual, without worrying about crippling flare ups.

I hope that you enjoyed this book, and if you did, feel free to leave a review. Thank you.

Description

Are you suffering from chronic inflammation that hinders your every day life? Well you are not alone. Millions of people around the world find themselves fighting inflammation on a daily basis. The good news is that there is hope to be had. You can simply change your diet, and you will find an improved life.

This book will show you exactly how to do that. So what are you waiting for? Enjoy this book, and start living your life without inflammation again.

www.ingramcontent.com/pod-product-compliance
Lightning Source LLC
Chambersburg PA
CBHW071249280526
45788CB00004B/1640